Hypertension Down Naturally

My Research, Findings & Success!

A 31 Day Meal Plan to Freedom

7 Potent & Tested Natural Remedies

By

Rick Robinson

Published by:

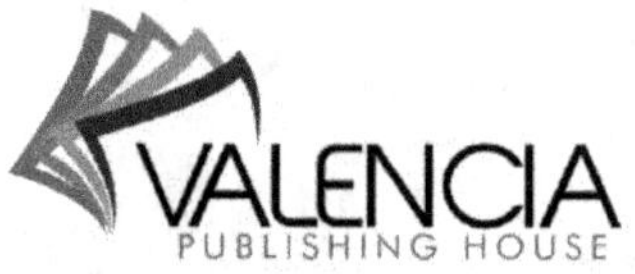

Valencia Publishing House

Cover & Interior designed

By

Rebecca Floyd

First Edition

WHAT'S IN THIS BOOK

High blood pressure is a serious, treatable and a wholly avoidable medical scourge that afflicts anywhere between 67 and 75 million Americans. Current medical research studies suggest that barely one-half of all people who are afflicted with high blood pressure problems are aware of it and take proactive and concerted steps to control it. This is another reason why high blood pressure is such a serious medical condition – most people who have high blood pressure are not even aware of it. Not until it is usually too late.

It has been estimated via medical research and study that over one thousand people afflicted with high blood pressure die because of it, or through medical conditions related to it, every single day. High blood pressure has no outwardly recognizable symptoms. In this manner, high blood pressure can truly be called a silent killer.

However, it doesn't have to be this way at all. For most people, high blood pressure is an extremely avoidable medical problem. High blood pressure, which is also known as hypertension, can be a wholly hereditary medical condition for some people. Still, high blood pressure is manifested and worsened by physical inactivity, lack of exercise and poor dietary lifestyle choices. Medical problems related to high blood pressure do not occur overnight. It can take a lot of time for high blood pressure to wreak havoc on the human body.

This means that you have the power to control it, maintain it and even reverse some of the damage that high blood pressure can cause. However, you have to know that you have high blood pressure in the first place. You have to act early. You should get medically checked out at least once a year, if not every six months. Most important of all, you must decide to take control over your exercise and dietary lifestyle. Always exercise regularly and eat a healthy, balanced diet.

When you take care of your body, your body will take care of you. Also, your heart will take care of you. Your heart is a muscle, and it is the most vital muscle that you possess within your body. High blood pressure, over time, can damage your heart and the blood vessels that serve it beyond all repair and hope. However, you should still remember the operative word in the previous sentence – *time.* If you know you have high blood pressure early enough, you should be able to reverse, or at least appreciably reduce, its effects.

(1 *"High Blood Pressure Facts."* https://www.cdc.gov/bloodpressure/facts.htm)

Take care of your body, exercise and eat right and you may not develop high blood pressure at all. Time is always on your side. That is if you learn you have high blood pressure early enough.

The odd thing about general public awareness when it comes to high blood pressure is that, as mentioned before, most people aren't even aware that they have high blood pressure. Some people may be aware of the term and may not even know what, "blood pressure," means even is as a medical term. Well, you need to know that this is OK. Human beings learn something new every day.

It is OK if you don't know what blood pressure is. What is not OK, is not endeavoring to learn as much as you can about high blood pressure as soon as possible. Almost 360,000 people died in the United States in the year 2013 due to high blood pressure or via symptoms and medical conditions related to it. That number must go down to zero as much as possible because high blood pressure is avoidable and reversible. Education is the key.

People are more susceptible to the dangers of high blood pressure as we and our bodies' age. Being uninformed is not a crime, but being steadfastly and willfully ignorant can wind up being a crime to your health and heart. Honestly, your body may not survive the punishment that high blood pressure has in store for it.

In this book, you will learn about blood pressure, the dangers of high blood pressure and what high blood pressure can do to your body. You will learn about some of the medications and natural remedies that you can use to combat high blood pressure and keep your blood pressure under control.

You will also learn about the importance of exercise, keeping a food diary and adopting a healthier eating lifestyle. In this book, you will also find a sample, thirty-one-day healthy food menu that you can use to model your own food diary after.

In this book, you will learn everything that you need to learn about healthily getting on your way to maintaining your blood pressure. Remember that being informed, educated and having time on your side is the key.

So, let's take it from the beginning. What exactly is blood pressure?

BLOOD PRESSURE

While it is in no way an exact analogy, it helps to think about blood pressure in a similar way to a 10-story apartment building. Imagine that your heart is an apartment on the fifth floor. All of the pipes and plumbing that connect water to your apartment in this hypothetical building can be compared to arteries and veins. If the water pressure in the pipes in your building is extremely too high, then water will shoot out of the faucets at high speed of velocity.

This will corrode, crack and weaken pipes. Even damage or destroy them. If the water pressure is extremely too low, then no water will reach your apartment. It is not an exact analogy, but good enough to scratch the surface of explaining blood pressure in the human body.

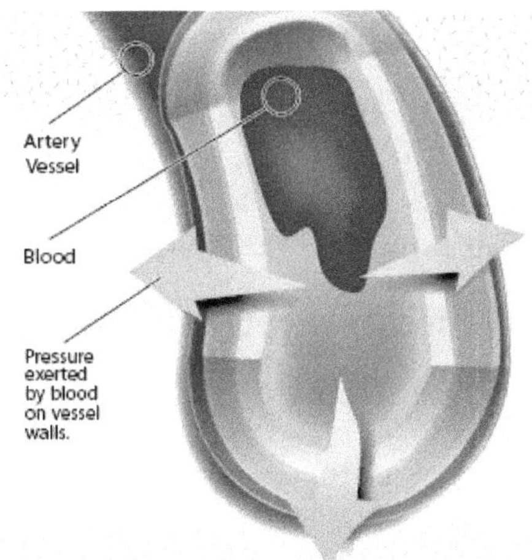

What is blood pressure?

Blood pressure is the force that moves blood through your arteries. Arteries are the blood vessels that carry blood from your heart to the rest of your body. High blood pressure is when your blood pressure is usually higher than it should be. It is also called **hypertension.**

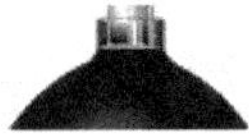

(Sources: FDA.gov)

Your heart pushes blood out to its arteries with every heartbeat. Blood flows throughout your body based on the force of your heart pushing and propelling it through your arteries and blood vessels via heartbeats. "Blood pressure," refers to the amount of force that is exerted against the walls of your arteries as blood is ferried through the blood vessels. Veins are blood vessels that ferry oxygen-starved blood to the heart to be re-oxygenized, and those blood vessels are propelled by blood pressure from the heart as well.

It is imperative that the blood pressure flowing against the walls of the blood vessels within your body do so continuously and at a normal rate of speed. On the average, your heart pumps and propels blood through your blood vessels by beating about 60 to 70 times a minute, more or less. Your blood pressure is at its peak, or it's highest when the heart is forcefully pumping out blood during a heartbeat. This is known as your systolic blood pressure. The exact moment in time between your heart beatings, when your heart is momentarily at rest, is what is known as your diastolic blood pressure.

If you have ever had your blood pressure taken, then you know that a doctor or nurse checks your blood pressure by wrapping an inflatable cuff device around your arm. This device is formally known as a sphygmomanometer. This inflatable cuff device inflates with air, almost like a balloon, and squeezes your arm. In reality, this inflatable arm cuff device is squeezing the blood vessels within your arm and measuring the speed at which your blood flows through the blood vessels in your arm. It is also measuring the force of the blood pressure that is being exerted against the walls of your blood vessels within your arm.

Your blood pressure is visualized to you in two numbers. Normal blood pressure readings are usually just under 120/80, or, "120 over 80." This number is the baseline for normal blood pressure. Your blood pressure should be near it or just under it a little. The first number is your systolic blood pressure reading and the second number is your diastolic blood pressure reading. If your blood pressure reading is ever over 140/90, then you have high blood pressure.

If your blood pressure readings are ever in the range of 180/120, then you have what is called a "hypertensive emergency crisis," and need to be hospitalized immediately. Such a dire systolic over diastolic blood pressure reading would mean that your blood pressure is racing and propelling blood dangerously through your blood vessels. Also, your blood pressure would be exerting such a pressure against the walls of your blood vessels that your body, and the organs within your body, would not be able to cope for long.

A blood pressure reading of 90/60 and anything under is considered to be too low. Low blood pressure can cause fainting spells, blackouts, dizziness, and feelings of nausea. Low blood pressure can cause the body to cease functioning because blood is not reaching any organs at all. The brain can seize or stroke with high blood pressure. However, with low blood pressure, the brain may not get enough or any blood replenishment at all, which is highly dangerous as well.

(Source: Heart.org)

So, there you have it. That, in a nutshell, is a basic rundown of what blood pressure is and how important it is to bodily function. Remember, a healthy blood pressure reading is just under 120/80.

The best way to avoid the dangers of high blood pressure is to be as informed as possible about the dangers it can impose upon your body. There are just too many ways for high blood pressure to wreck medical havoc upon your body. After all, it is a silent killer for a reason. So, let's talk about the numerous medical dangers that are associated with high blood pressure.

Being as educated and informed as possible about the dangers of high blood pressure is highly important.

To put it bluntly, it is not the high blood pressure within itself that will kill you. You can live with high blood pressure and not even know it for years and decades. It's the effects that high blood pressure will have on your body that will kill you.

Imagine that you open your sink or bathtub faucets and water shoots out of it at high speed of velocity. Such highly intense water pressure is bound to cause many problems with the internal plumbing of our hypothetical apartment building. If the apartment on the fifth floor of our hypothetical building represent your heart, and the water is shooting out of all of the faucets, then imagine how inefficiently the water pressure is in reaching other apartments in the building.

Imagine that the other apartments in the building represent your organs and limbs. That is the problem with high blood pressure in your body. It makes your heart work harder than it needs to. High blood pressure can also dangerously weaken your heart. High blood pressure can also affect how efficiently blood is ferried to other organs and other parts of the body.

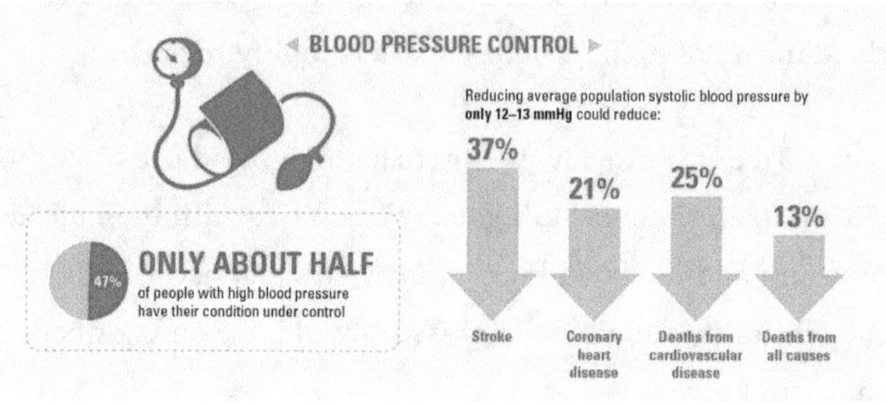

(Source: CDC.gov)

As I mentioned earlier, there are just too many ways for high blood pressure to wreak havoc on the human body. High blood pressure shows no outward symptoms, so you may not even realize that you have it. Not until it is too late anyway. Time is your ally with high blood pressure.

The earlier that you know you have high blood pressure, the more time that you have to possibly reverse its effects. High blood pressure can take months, years or even decades in some people to cause serious medical problems. Sometimes, the medical damage caused by high blood pressure can be irreparable and irreversible, especially if you learn you have it too late to do anything about it.

High blood pressure can cause you to develop a host of medical problems. Let's examine some of them.

8 MAJOR HEALTH RISKS FROM HYPERTENSION

BLOOD VESSEL CONSTRICTION

High blood pressure can constrict or severely, and dangerously, narrow the blood vessels circulating throughout your body. This means that there is less blood floating through your blood vessels. This means that less blood is being ferried by blood vessels to your organs. Constricted blood vessels can also cause the dangerous accumulation of calcium and plaque within them, which can also cause artery clogging and/or a pileup of blood cells or blood clots.

A blood clot is a gel-like or partially-solid mass of blood that is helpful in repairing injuries. High blood pressure can also cause blood cells and/or blood clots to become wedged and trapped in constricted blood vessels. This situation can deprive the heart, brain, and body in general, of desperately needed blood. This can cause a heart attack or stroke. Be aware that a stroke can happen in your heart or your brain tissue.

CORONARY HEART DISEASE

High blood pressure, which can be a hereditary condition, is also a leading factor to cause coronary heart disease. Coronary arteries are the blood vessels responsible for supplying the heart directly with oxygen-rich blood. With this disease, calcium and/or plaque slowly builds up and accumulates within the coronary arteries. Like a clogged pipe under a sink or in the wall of an apartment. The calcium and /or plaque accumulation can block blood flow over time, or further enable a blood clot or mass of blood cells to accelerate a clogged blockage in the coronary artery. High blood pressure will steadily accelerate and worsen, this condition over years or even decades.

Blood racing through blood vessels at a high velocity can also weaken, rot and decay the walls of your blood vessels. In this manner, high blood pressure can cause internal hemorrhaging. Imagine a water pipe bursting in the walls of your building. All that water can cause rot, mold, and weakening of the structure.

High blood pressure, coupled with obesity, physical inactivity, not exercising regularly, poor diet and eating food rich in fat, can also lead to the development of diabetes.

ANEURYSM

You can easily develop an aneurysm if you have high blood pressure. An aneurysm is an abnormal, protruding bulge in an artery or blood vessel that can resemble a balloon. High blood pressure can cause this abnormal, stretched out protrusion of the blood vessel.

An aneurysm isn't fatal within itself; it is the tendency for it to burst without notice that makes it deadly. An aortic aneurysm is a burst blood vessel that can cause internal bleeding or hemorrhage within the heart. A cerebral aneurysm is the same problem happening within the brain. There are many kinds of aneurysms, but these two can be fatal if high blood pressure is left unchecked.

ENLARGED HEART

You can develop an abnormally enlarged heart with sustained and untreated high blood pressure medical issues. A weakened, enlarged heart cannot pump blood efficiently. Blood will have to pump out harder and faster with an enlarged heart. The more effort exerted by an enlarged heart, the more that it is weakened. An enlarged heart cannot serve the organs upon which a steady flow of blood is dependent on for proper functioning. An enlarged heart is a weakened heart, and a weakened heart is destined to fail over time.

If you have an enlarged heart and high blood pressure problems, then you are over four times as likely to have a heart attack as someone with a normal-sized heart.

KIDNEY FAILURE

Did you know that your kidneys can fail if you have untreated high blood pressure issues? Your kidneys produce a hormone that helps to regulate your blood pressure. Your kidneys also function as a waste filter that helps to clean and purify your blood. Your kidneys also function to remove bodily fluid waste from your body, as well as excess fluids.

Your heart pumps blood to all of the organs in your body, including your kidneys. If your blood vessels, or arteries, become constricted and narrowed, then this can cause damage to your kidneys. Not enough blood will reach it and will steadily weaken it. Your kidneys produce a hormone called aldosterone which helps to regulate your body's internal blood pressure.

(2 *"Blood Pressure and You."*

www.bloodpressureuk.org/BloodPressureandyou/Yourbody/Enlargedheart)

If you have high blood pressure, then your kidneys can't produce the hormone which can correct the problem, which can result in a downward spiral of overlapping medical problems.

The kidneys are also instrumental in filtering waste from your blood. If you have high blood pressure, then the blood in your blood vessels is being propelled too fast to be cleaned properly. This means that your unfiltered, polluted and oxygen-starved blood will be ferried throughout your body, damaging other organs. What's worse, the more that your kidney is damaged, the less your blood will be filtered. This can lead to the need for dialysis or the external, mechanical cleaning of blood. Or even the need for a kidney transplant.

STRESS

Medical research suggests that stress and prolonged emotional tension can increase high blood pressure in the short term. When you are angry and incredibly stressed, the human body releases a surge of hormones that compel the heart to beat rapidly and for your blood pressure to increase.

It will take a very long time for stress to cause medical damage, but stress is a real silent killer that enables and empowers high blood pressure. If you are stressed out and angry for long period of time, then the walls of your arteries and blood vessels will steadily and incrementally become damaged by high blood pressure.

BLINDNESS

Untreated high blood pressure can lead to blurred vision and/or complete loss of sight. There are a few ways that this can happen.

As mentioned before, high blood pressure can narrow and constrict the blood vessels in your arteries and blood vessels throughout the body. If the blood flow to the blood vessels that serve the eyes, also known as capillaries, are restricted in a significant way, then blurry vision or complete vision loss can be the result. If your high blood pressure causes a buildup of calcium and/or plaque in your blood vessels, which can block blood flow, you can have a stroke. If the blood flow to your eyes is blocked, this can damage or destroy the optic nerves in your eyes. Partial or complete blindness will follow. So, always keep in mind that one of the best ways to protect your eyes and vision is to know about and healthily maintain your blood pressure.

SEVERE BONE DENSITY LOSS

Untreated and prolonged high blood pressure can cause a significant increase in calcium to be deposited in your urine and the muscular cells in your body instead of your bones. Your bones require calcium to grow, become dense and to be stronger. Calcium loss via high blood pressure is a leading factor in the development of osteoporosis, a medical condition where your bones become very fragile due to extreme calcium loss and deficiency.

If you have osteoporosis, your bones can become so brittle that you can break or fracture your wrist trying to open a jar. Osteoporosis is prone to afflict middle-aged and elderly women a lot more than other people.

The medical conditions that were just mentioned are barely the tip of the iceberg when it comes to the problems that high blood pressure that can induce within the human body Remember, it's not the high blood pressure within itself that will kill you. It's the symptoms and medical problems caused by high blood pressure that will kill you.

You may be able to live with high blood pressure problems for years or decades. It is all of the various medical problems that high blood pressure can cause you, and in your body, which will kill you.

It pays to be as informed about your risk for high blood pressure as much as possible. Always remember, time is on your side if you get medically checked out and learn if you are at risk for high blood pressure early enough.

There are numerous factors that can contribute to the development of high blood pressure. High blood pressure is a genetically hereditary condition that can be passed down several family generations. You may develop high blood pressure through no fault of your own and be entirely unaware of it.

That fact, however, does not absolve you from the responsibility of getting regularly checked out for high blood pressure. Being informed and educated is the key to surviving the threat of high blood pressure.

You may have high blood pressure if you are...

The more areas that describe you, the greater the chance that you may have high blood pressure now or in the future.

A smoker
Dealing with sleep apnea
Physically inactive
Older than 50 years
Overweight or obese
Dealing with diabetes or kidney disease
Taking more than 2 grams of sodium per day
African American, Hispanic or Latino/Latina
A man who drinks more than 1 ounce of alcohol per day
A woman who drinks more than half an ounce of alcohol per day
A person whose mother or father has hypertension

(Source: FDA.gov)

ETHNICITY

Several medical studies have also suggested that race and ethnicity can play a significant factor in identifying exactly who is more prone to develop high blood pressure over others. People of African and Asian races and ethnicities have been medically researched and documented to suffer from high blood pressure more than other races. Some studies suggest that African Americans, in particular, are much more susceptible to the ravages of high blood pressure than any other race or ethnicity. **3** Such factors can be negated, however, by heredity, obesity, sedentary and physically inactive lifestyles and bad diet.

OLD AGE

You can be at risk to develop high blood pressure due to the unstoppable onslaught of old age. As we the age, the human body cellularly breaks down. Internal organs, like the heart, can become older and more worn down after decades of operation.

(3 *"Know Your Risk Factors for High Blood Pressure."*
www.heart.org/HEARTORG/Conditions/HighBloodPressure/UnderstandYourRis

Arteries and blood vessels can harden and constrict naturally with the advance of time.

Our blood vessels also become appreciably less elastic as we age. That doesn't mean that all hope is lost, however. You can counter these effects as much as possible with regular exercise and adopting a healthier eating lifestyle.

OBESITY

Being morbidly obese raises your chances of developing high blood pressure significantly. If you are severely overweight, then you may be twice as likely to develop high blood pressure as someone who is not. When you are overweight, you cause your heart, blood vessels in your body and your entire circulatory system to work a lot more than it should need to. Obesity can strain the heart and cause it to become abnormally enlarged. An enlarged heart is a weakened heart.

Find out your body mass index, the metric upon which you can learn your optimal weight, exercise regularly and eat healthier. Ask your doctor to tell you your exact BMI measurement.

SMOKING

The act of smoking cigarettes increases your heart rate and appreciably raises your blood pressure. Smoking also narrows or constricts your blood vessels. Smoking also causes calcium and plaque to accumulate in your blood vessels. High blood pressure can doubly accelerate the rate at which smoking-induced calcium and plaque can accumulate in your blood vessels.

This process can occur even with the inhalation of nearby second-hand smoke. Each and every time that you smoke, you will temporarily increase your blood pressure rate. This adds up over time and can lead to stroke, heart attack, coronary heart disease or cancer.

The more that you smoke, the more that you will compound the problem, the threat of high blood pressure, over time. Stop smoking. Avoid secondhand smoke as much as possible.

ALCOHOL

Always drink moderately and responsibly, optimally less than two or three drinks per day. Excessive binge-like drinking over long periods can cause your blood pressure to appreciably rise to dangerous levels. Continued, excessive drinking over long period of time can cause long-term damage via high blood pressure.

PHYSICAL INACTIVITY

One of the best ways to combat the effects, or onset, of high blood pressure is to exercise regularly. You should exercise every day, if not every other day. Employ some repetitions of aerobic and resistance based exercise as much as possible. Try to find the time to exercise an accumulated 90 minutes to two and a half hours every week, if possible.

You don't have to endure high resistance weight training or Olympic caliber workout routines either. Ride a bike. Take the stairs instead of the elevator as much as possible. Walk as much as possible. Talk to your doctor about developing a custom exercise regimen that is right for you and your health needs.

UNHEALTHY DIETARY LIFESTYLE

Lower your sodium, or salt, intake considerably. Ingesting too much salt raises your blood pressure. It can also cause you to retain more fluid in your body than normal, which can increase blood pressure and strain your organs. This can cause your arteries and blood vessels to harden and constrict considerably, increasing your chance of a stroke or an aneurysm.

Too much salt in your diet can also cause your kidneys to become severely strained and damaged. Your kidneys filter your blood and release hormones that help to regulate your blood pressure. Your kidneys work hard enough filtering and cleaning your blood. If there is too much salt in your body, then your kidneys must work overtime to filter the excess salt along with the impurities and waste in your body. Over time, this overstrain of work will greatly and appreciably interfere with the kidney's role in regulating your body's blood pressure as well as filtering your blood.

Eating unhealthy food that is high in fat, trans fatty acids like those found in fried foods, cholesterol and calories will result in obesity and the need for the human body to work harder to function. This will lead to high blood pressure which can lead to constricted blood vessels, stroke, heart attack and coronary heart disease. Adopting a healthier eating lifestyle is the best way to ward off high blood pressure and all of the medical issues that it can cause you.

There are many ways that you can become at-risk to develop high blood pressure. As I will keep mentioning, the best defense against high blood pressure is to be as educated and informed about it as humanly possible.

HOW TO PREVENT HIGH BLOOD PRESSURE

There are several ways that you can prevent high blood pressure. The best way is to be informed about your own blood pressure health. Get medically checked out regularly, or at least once a year. Find out your blood pressure numbers. Ask your doctor or medical professional what you can do to improve your blood pressure numbers and maintain them at a healthy level.

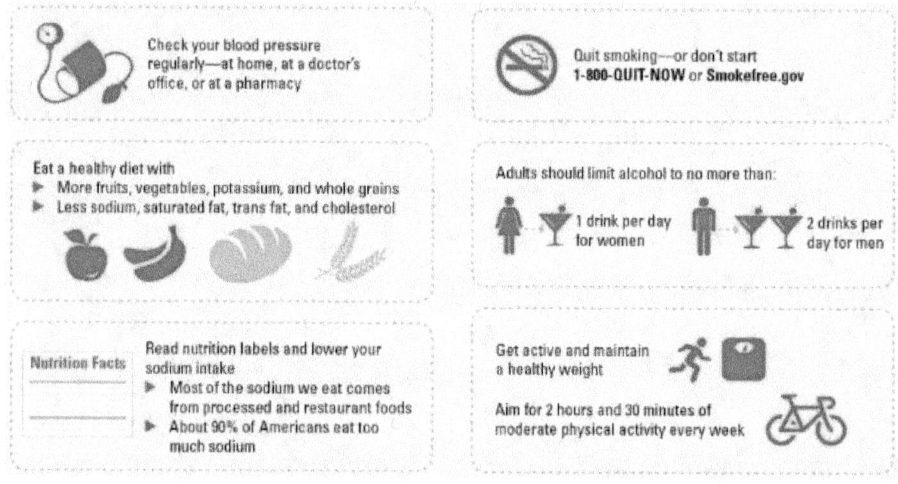

(**Source:** Naturalon.com)

Here is a listing of just a few things you can do on your own to prevent the onset of high blood pressure.

EXERCISE REGULARLY

The best way to prevent the onset of high blood pressure is to exercise and to maintain a healthy body weight. Learn your exact body mass index number from your doctor. Your body mass index, or BMI, is a metric that will tell you how much body fat that you should have on your body and what your ideal or optimum body weight should be.

Everyone's body mass index is distinct and unique. If you are obese, or severely overweight, then you will cause considerable strain on your body, and its interior organs, just to function properly.

Put simply, if you are obese, then you are twice as likely to develop high blood pressure as someone who is not obese. Exercise as much as you can. You can exercise every day or every other day. However, it is important that you make regular, consistent thirty-minute exercise routines a permanent part of your personal lifestyle.

STOP SMOKING

Do not smoke. If you don't smoke, don't find reasons to start. It is not worth the significant damage that it will do to your body or your blood pressure health. If you have a hard time trying to quit, ask your doctor for help.

Continued and prolonged periods of smoking will severely narrow, or constrict, your arteries and blood vessels over time. You raise your blood pressure incrementally every time that you smoke. This will take a toll on your blood pressure health over years and decades, to a point where the damage will become irreversible.

LIMIT SALT INTAKE

Remove salt from your diet or use it as little and sparingly as possible. Try to limit your salt intake to 1,500 to 2,300 milligrams daily, if possible. For the sake of reference, 2,300 milligrams is just about equal to one teaspoon of salt.

Try to limit the amount of cured luncheon meats that you consume, as those are loaded with salt for preserving and flavoring purposes. Experiment with salt substitutes and other spices and learn to use those to substitute for salt.

Limit the amount of fried and fast foods that you eat. Examine the ingredients of the processed foods that you eat. A lot of those, like instant ramen, are full of salt, also known as sodium.

Over the long term, large intakes of salt can do significant destructive damage to your kidneys and increase your high blood pressure. If you want to control, maintain or reverse your high blood pressure, you are going to have to learn how to live without salt. Or learn how to live with eating much less of it.

LIMIT DAILY ALCOHOL INTAKE

Consume three or less alcoholic drinks daily. You increase your blood pressure incrementally with every sip and drink of alcohol. Seek help from your doctor or medical professional if you think you have a drinking problem.

USE THE D.A.S.H. DIET

The Dietary Approaches to Stop Hypertension, or the D.A.S.H. Diet, is a dietary plan that is designed to help lower high blood pressure in the long term in conjunction with regular exercise. The Dash Diet is mainly composed of foods that are extremely low-fat, non-dairy, rich in fiber, calcium, potassium, and magnesium and comprised of a lot of fruits and vegetables.

With the D.A.S.H. Diet, you will consume a lot of nuts, legumes, seeds and whole grains. With this diet, it is important to eat lean, low-fatty cuts of protein and a lot of fish. You should take all skin off poultry meats before consuming them. It is also nutritionally and vitally important broil, bake, roast or grill all your protein meats instead of unhealthily frying them.

You are allowed to use frying oil with the D.A.S.H. Diet, but it should be in minute amounts, like one tablespoon or less. You should only use cooking oils rich in monounsaturated and polyunsaturated fats. Such oils include canola oil, corn oil, olive oil, vegetable oil, peanut oil and soybean oil.

You should consume vegetables that are raw and have not been processed. Such vegetables contain more amounts of fiber. Fruit will be a large part of your diet with this plan as well since they are high in potassium, magnesium, and fiber. Grains, bread, pasta, rice and other carbohydrate sources should be eaten at a minimum, like a half a cup daily or less.

According to medical research studies conducted by the National Heart Lung and Blood Institute, people who employ the D.A.S.H. Diet with consistent, regular exercise can see their systolic blood pressure numbers reduced by over 11 points and their diastolic blood pressure numbers reduced by over 5 points over a two-week period.

The DASH (Dietary Approaches to Stop Hypertension) diet can help you control your blood pressure. It's not just about keeping your sodium intake low. It's about finding the right combination of sodium plus nutrients like potassium, magnesium and calcium. You can get these nutrients by eating lots of fruits and vegetables, low-fat dairy products and lean animal products.

Here is an example of a 2,000-calorie DASH diet plan:*

Food Group	Number of Servings per Day
Grains & breads	7-8
Vegetables	4-5
Fruits	4-5
Low-fat/nonfat dairy	2-3
Meat, poultry, fish	6 ounces or less
Nuts, seeds, dry beans	4-5 per week

* Depending on your weight, height, gender, age and activity level, your calorie needs may differ.

(Source: Clevelandclinic.org)

(4 *"Eating Well To Lower Your Blood Pressure."*
http://chfs.ky.gov/NR/rdonlyres/5D24E0C9-3602-404D-AFDC-A7195B2BDD5F/0/DASHDIET.pdf)

The D.A.S.H Diet was developed for daily, 2,000 calories dietary meal plans. The D.A.S.H Diet is not a cure for high blood pressure, but it can be used as a key in helping you maintain it.

It has been stressed that a large part of fighting high blood pressure is to be as educated and as informed as possible. While that is true, it may not always be enough. You also have to be proactive, eat right, take care of your body and get your blood pressure checked out regularly. Be informed, but take all of the necessary action that you need to reduce your blood pressure. Your health and your life may depend on it.

BLOOD PRESSURE MEDICATIONS

In this section, I will give you a general overview of the kinds of medications that are usually prescribed to people with high blood pressure. If you go for a medical check-up, get your blood pressure checked and your doctor suggests prescribing medication to treat it, then your high blood pressure has reached an unstable point. Especially so when medication must be used to treat it.

This book should not be used as a substitute for the medical advice given to you by a doctor or medical professional. Always trust your doctor. The information given to you in this book should be used for informational purposes only.

As previously mentioned, when you have come to the point where you need medication to control and maintain your blood pressure, then you can be assured that you have moderate to extremely serious issues with your blood pressure. If you have to take medication to control and maintain your blood pressure, then executing extreme and consistent lifestyle and dietary changes may just not be enough anymore.

Always take your medication exactly as prescribed by your doctor. Also, remember that medicinal dosages for high blood pressure are different and unique to each person. The details for the treatment of your high blood pressure medication regimen will depend on your health, medical history and how well you take care of your body.

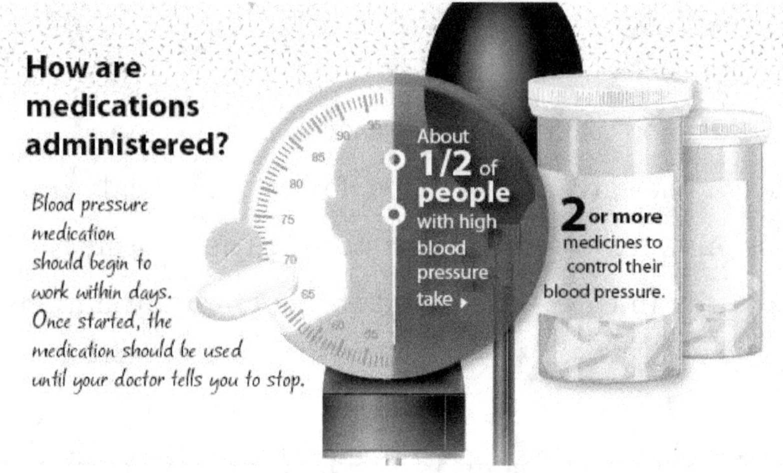

(Source: FDA.gov)

There are literally thousands of kinds of high blood pressure alleviating medications on the open market. I will mention a couple of the most common ones that your doctor might prescribe to you to help you maintain your high blood pressure.

THIAZIDE DIURETICS

Thiazide diuretics are more generally known as, "water pills." As we have discussed before, high blood pressure can cause significant renal, or kidney damage. The kidneys filter your blood and also help to regulate your blood pressure. High blood pressure can cause severe narrowing, or constriction, of blood vessels.

Constricted blood vessels can cause less blood to reach the kidneys, damaging them, their ability to regulate blood pressure and filter blood as well. If you ingest too much salt, you can also cause your blood vessels to become constricted as well as overload your kidneys with work. Your kidneys will now have to work overtime to filter out excess salt as well as purify your blood. Over time, this will cause significant damage to your kidneys.

Diuretics are designed to help your kidneys work better. Diuretics help your kidneys remove salt, excess water and fluid from your blood quicker and more efficiently. This process will reduce overall blood volume and require less force to generate against the walls of your blood vessels.

If there are less salt and excess fluid in your bloodstream, then your heart does not have to work hard to propel blood throughout your circulatory system. This will help to reduce your blood pressure.

BETA BLOCKERS

Beta blockers are a kind of high blood pressure medication that are designed to reduce the workload exerted by your heart when it pumps blood throughout your circulatory system. Once ingested, beta blockers will slowly and safely reduce the rate of your heartbeats.

If your heart beats with less force, then it will generate less force as it pumps blood. In turn, your blood pressure will incrementally become lower. Beta blockers are extremely potent pharmaceutical drugs. You should take this medication exactly as directed by your doctor.

CALCIUM CHANNEL BLOCKERS

Calcium channel blockers are designed to relax and help slowly widen constricted blood vessels. Their main function is the prevention of calcium being deposited in the cells of the heart and within your blood vessels. When calcium enters the cells of the heart and blood vessels, they cause harder and forceful contractions to occur, which in turn increases blood pressure. Calcium deposits in your blood vessels will also cause clogged blockages in your bloodstream sooner or later.

ACE INHIBITORS

Ace inhibitors are a class of drugs that are designed to reduce the production of a harmful chemical within the human body. The chemical angiotensin, when produced naturally in the human body, causes blood vessels to narrow and constrict. The "ACE," in ACE inhibitor stands for, "angiotensin-converting enzyme," formally. ACE inhibitors block the generation of angiotensin which in turn helps reduce the narrowing of blood vessels.

BLOOD THINNERS

The term, "blood thinner," is a bit of misnomer. Blood thinners do not actually, "thin," out your blood. Blood thinners are more formally known as anticoagulants. Anticoagulants reduces the blood's ability to form blood clots. If you have narrowed, constricted arteries that are filled with calcium and plaque deposits, then a blood thinner will reduce your chances of developing a stroke or heart attack.

Blood thinners primarily prevent your narrowed arteries and blood vessels from becoming blocked and clogged by calcium, plaque or blood clots. While blood thinners are useful in this regard in alleviating the effects of high blood pressure, they can also be dangerous if not taken exactly as prescribed.

If you are ever severely cut or physically injure yourself while taking a blood thinner, then your blood will not clot, or clot effectively enough to slow down severe bleeding. You could bleed to death. So, use this medication exactly as prescribed by your doctor.

There are literally thousands of kinds of high blood pressure medications that are prescribed to patients every year. These are just a few of the more generally recognized medications. The medication that you are prescribed by your doctor will depend upon your present health condition, family history and how well you take care of your body.

Also remember that if you have to take medication as prescribed by your doctor, then your high blood pressure problems have become very serious. Always follow your doctor's directions.

31-DAY MAINTENANCE GUIDE AND DIETARY MENU PLAN

This a daily high blood pressure maintenance guide to help you keep your blood pressure under control. Think of this as a blood pressure management guide for your dietary needs. As you should be vitally aware, food, exercise, and lifestyle adjustment play a big role in blood pressure maintenance. In fact, exercise and diet play the most important part of any lifestyle change you personally adopt.

You can follow this high blood pressure maintenance guide for exercise and dietary needs exactly. Or you can use it as a basic template to suit your own needs.

This high blood pressure maintenance guide was developed to help reinforce the need for lifestyle changes. If you have high blood pressure problems, you must now always take into consideration what you eat. You have to think about whether or not the food you eat will worsen or help alleviate your high blood pressure.

The most important lifestyle change that you should adopt is learning to exercise every day or at least every other day. As we have previously discussed, inactivity worsens high blood pressure problems. Whether or not you have been prescribed medication to fight the effects of high blood pressure, nothing should exempt you from adjusting your personal lifestyle to accommodate regular, moderate and low-impact exercise.

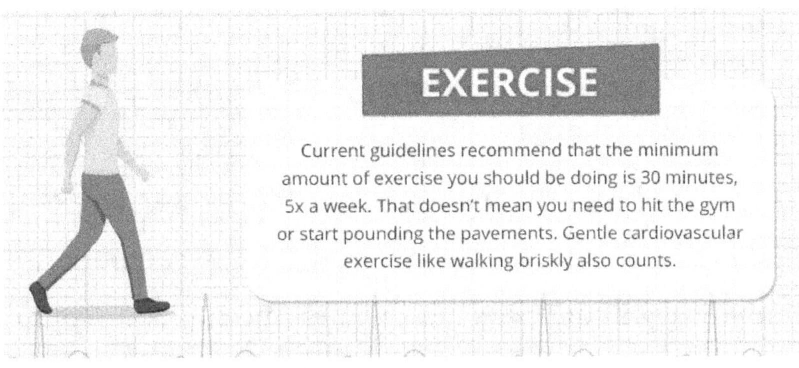

(**Source:** Wellman Clinic)

It is just not enough to be informed and educated about high blood pressure, especially if you have to take medication to maintain its effects. You must be proactive. Too many people have high blood pressure and aren't even aware of it because high blood pressure exhibits no outward symptoms at all.

In this next chapter you will find the 31-day meal and light exercise regimen that I tested and tried, and as I told you it worked for my family and friends, and I am confident, it will do the same for you. Do me a favor, give it a try and stay on it for at least 3 weeks before you knock it.

But before we get into the 31-day high blood pressure maintenance guide, let's talk about the need to keep a food diary.

FOOD DIARY

A food diary is just exactly what it sounds like. In a regular diary, you write about your feelings, emotions or commentary about personal events and happenings in your life.

With a food diary you must regularly, honestly and accurately account for every calorie of food that you eat every day. Most people are so set in their ways, and used to high fat foods and convenient fast food, that they may not even think about what they eat or how much they eat.

From breakfast, lunch, dinner and every snack in between, write down and describe what you ate. Describe the meal, the portion and how long it took you to consume it. "Comfort food," is called comfort food for a reason. We eat what makes us feel good, without considering the caloric or health consequences to our bodies. Human beings tend to live to eat, instead of eating to live, especially Americans and the love of fast food culture.

When you keep an honest and accurate food diary, you will be made unequivocally aware of your eating habits and whether or not your eating habits are damaging your health. It is very hard to shrink from the truth. Especially when you find out that your own actions may be making your own health much worse.

Start keeping a food diary. When you do this, you will have confronted your own dietary consumptions actions and will have to decide what you must do to help alleviate your own high blood pressure problems.

KNOWING WHAT YOU EAT MATTERS

If you eat, "junk food," well, what do you think doing such will do to your body. You get whatever you put into your body.

It just doesn't make any sense to eat food that will damage your health or expedite the narrowing of your blood vessels.

The human cardiovascular system is significantly helped by the ingestion of low fat and low cholesterol diet. Lowering your cholesterol, by regularly eating food that are low in cholesterol, will greatly decrease the strain of high blood pressure on your circulatory system. Fiber refers to vegetables, good carbs and fruits. Foods that are rich in fiber also help make digestion go smoother as well as enable the endocrine systems in your body work better. The endocrine system is a system of glands located throughout the human body that releases hormones for various reason into the bloodstream to be ferried towards other organs.

Of course, you know that you must eat well to better combat high blood pressure. However, it is also important to know why you have to eat well.

WHAT TO BUY AT THE SUPERMARKET?

HIGH BLOOD PRESSURE MAINTENANCE SHOPPING LIST

Carrots, Corn, star fruit

Parsnips, Red Potatoes, pumpkin

Golden potatoes, Fennel, pear

Leafy Greens, Spinach, papaya

Beets, Red cabbage, avocado

Napa cabbage, Bok Choy, plums

Brussels sprouts, Radish, peaches

Kale, Cress, sweet peas

Mustard Greens, Turnips, raspberries

Endive, Broccoli, strawberries

Arugula, Turnip Greens, blueberries

Chive, Green onion, dragon fruit

Peas, Water chestnuts, mango

Swiss chard, Wheatgrass, watermelons

Miners lettuce, Green beans, cantaloupe

Italian green beans, Pea pods, blackberries

French green beans, Cucumbers, honeydew

Cauliflower, Peppers, banana, Crowder peas

Eggplants, Zucchini, cherries

Yellow squash, Sweet potatoes, grapes

Artichokes, Taro, kiwi

Rutabaga, Rhubarb, star fruit

Okra, Tomatillo, grapefruit

Green tomatoes, White tomatoes

Kohlrabi, Snow peas, orange

Edamame, pea pods, lemon

Radish, Garlic, tangerine

Leek, Chicory, apples

Shallot, Chayote, Asian pear

Yacon, Maca, jackfruit

Okra, Ollusa. Limes

Mashua, Wasabi

Daikon, Horseradish

Salsify, Bitter Melon, Red Tomato

Sunchokes, Patty Pans Squash green

New Zealand Spinach, Spaghetti Squash

Acorn Squash, Yellow Squash

Raw Almonds

Cayenne Pepper (dried ground)

Raw Apple cider vinegar

DAY 1

EXERCISE

Daily exercise regimen can include brisk, 20-minute walking

MORNING MENU

Meat or Protein: Eggs and cheese

Carbohydrates: Half of a bran muffin

Drink: Water and a small coffee

Fruits and Vegetables: Half a cup to a full cup of Carrots, Corn and star fruit

SNACK MENU

Meat or Protein: Unsalted and non-roasted almonds and cheese

Carbohydrates: Half of a bagel

Drink: Water

Fruits and Vegetables: Miners lettuce, green beans and half of a cantaloupe

---

LUNCH MENU

Meat or Protein: Grilled chicken (Breast or thighs)

Carbohydrates: Half a cup of roasted red potatoes

Drink: Water and tea

Fruits and Vegetable: Carrots, Corn, and star fruit

SNACK MENU

Meat or Protein: Half a cup of bean

Carbohydrates: Cornbread muffin

Drink: Water

Fruits and Vegetables: Italian green beans, Pea pods, and blackberries with plain yogurt

---

DINNER MENU

Meat or Protein: Broiled turkey

Carbohydrates: Half a cup of unsalted stuffing

Drink: Water and coffee or tea

Fruits and Vegetable: Leafy Greens, Spinach, and papaya fruit

EXERCISE

Daily exercise includes a 20-minute to 30-minute walk on the treadmill or around the neighborhood.

MORNING MENU

Meat or Protein: Half a can of water packed sardines

Carbohydrates: 1 cup of sticky rice

Drink: Water and decaffeinated coffee or Tea

Fruits and Vegetables: Half a cup to a full cup serving of blueberries and grapes with plain yogurt

SNACK MENU

Meat or Protein: Cheese and crackers

Carbohydrates: Half of a bagel

Drink: Water

Fruits and Vegetables: Green bean salad with kale lettuce

LUNCH MENU

Meat or Protein: Grilled turkey or chicken burger/sandwich

Carbohydrates: 2 slices of bread

Drink: Water and tea

Fruits and Vegetables: Lettuce, sliced cucumbers, and tomatoes

SNACK MENU

Meat or Protein: Black eye peas

Carbohydrates: Cornbread muffin

Drink: water

Fruits and Vegetables: Blackberries and plain yogurt

DINNER MENU

Meat or Protein: Roasted turkey

Carbohydrates: Bread dumplings

Drink: Water and red rooibos tea

Fruits and Vegetables: Papaya fruit salad

DAY 3

EXERCISE

Daily exercise: Resistance step training and squat-thrust workout for 30-minutes

MORNING MENU

Meat or Protein: Half of a can of water-packed sardines

Carbohydrates: About half a cup of sticky rice

Drink: A small cup of coffee

Fruits and Vegetables: Starfruit, blueberries, and plain yogurt

SNACK MENU

Meat or Protein: Half a cup of cream cheese

Carbohydrates: Half of a bagel

Drink: Water

Fruits and Vegetables: Half a cup of raspberries

LUNCH MENU

Meat or Protein: Quinoa veggie burger

Carbohydrates 2 slices of bread

Drink: Water and green tea

Fruits and Vegetable: Lettuce, tomato, and sliced zucchini

SNACK MENU

Meat or Protein: Half a cup of unsalted and non-fried peanuts/almonds

Carbohydrates: None

Drink: Water

Fruits and Vegetable: Green Papaya salad

DINNER MENU

Meat or Protein: Cottage cheese and two hard-boiled eggs

Carbohydrates: Cornbread

Drink: Water and tea

Fruits and Vegetable: Chef Salad with tomato, lettuce, and one-fourth of a cup of low-fat shredded cheese

DAY 4

EXERCISE

Daily exercise: Brisk power walk for half a mile.

MORNING MENU

Meat or Protein: Low-fat, skim-milk cheese omelet, and one poached egg

Carbohydrates: One slice of toast

Drink: Water and tea

Fruits and Vegetables: Half of cup of canned fruit cocktail salad

SNACK MENU

Meat or Protein: One-fourth of a cup of almonds

Carbohydrates: Half of one bagel

Drink: Water

Fruits and Vegetables: Half of a cup of grapes

LUNCH MENU

Meat or Protein: One skinless and broiled chicken thigh

Carbohydrates: half a cup of roasted potatoes

Drink: Water and tea

Fruits and Vegetables: Half a cup of corn

SNACK MENU

Meat or Protein: Half a cup of kidney beans

Carbohydrates: Cornbread muffin

Drink: Water

Fruits and Vegetables: Three bean salad

DINNER MENU

Meat or Protein: Baked chicken

Carbohydrates: Croutons with a sprinkling of shredded bacon

Drink: Water and tea

Fruits and Vegetables: Cesar salad

DAY 5

EXERCISE

Daily exercise: 30 minutes of moderate aerobic exercise.

MORNING MENU

Meat or Protein: Cheese omelet with lean steak strip

Carbohydrates: One bran muffin

Drinks: Water hot

Fruits and Vegetables: Two slices of watermelon

Meat or Protein: None

Carbohydrates: Half of one bagel

Drink: Water

Fruits and Vegetables: Half of a cup of unsweetened applesauce

LUNCH MENU

Meat or Protein: Roasted salmon fillet

Carbohydrates: Half a cup of roasted potatoes

Drink: Water and green tea

Fruits and Vegetables: One-fourth of a cup of baby carrots

SNACK MENU

Meat or Protein: Turkey soup

Carbohydrates: Cornbread

Drink: Water

Fruits and Vegetables: Italian green beans, pea pods, carrots

DINNER MENU

Meat or Protein: Mushroom soup with pieces of lean shredded meat

Carbohydrates: Two slices of multi-grain bread

Drink: Water and red rooibos tea

Fruits and Vegetables: Carrots and peas

DAY 6

EXERCISE

Daily exercise: 30 minutes of squat thrusts and jumping jacks

MORNING MENU

Meat or Protein: Turkey and Swiss cheese sandwich

Carbohydrates: One English muffin

Drink: Water and decaffeinated coffee

Fruits and Vegetables: Two bananas

SNACK MENU

Meat or Protein: Pistachios

Carbohydrates: One English muffin

Drink: Water

Fruits and Vegetables: Half a cup of blueberries with plain yogurt

---

LUNCH MENU

Meat or Protein: Poached salmon fillet

Carbohydrates: One cup of stuffing

Drink: Water and tea

Fruits and Vegetables: Stewed bok choy

SNACK MENU

Meat or Protein: Turkey soup with tomato sauce

Carbohydrates: Half a cup of tortellini pasta

Drink: Water

Fruits and Vegetables: Green beans, peas, carrots

DINNER MENU

Meat or Protein: Roasted turkey wings with pinto beans

Carbohydrates: Tortilla wrap

Drink: Water and Earl Grey tea

Fruits and Vegetables: spinach salad

DAY 7

EXERCISE

Daily exercise: 30 minutes of sit-ups, push-ups, jumping jacks and low impact aerobics

---

MORNING MENU

Meat or Protein: Low sodium turkey bacon and eggs

Carbohydrates: Half a cup of stuffing

Drink: Water and red rooibos tea

Fruits and Vegetables: One whole mango

SNACK MENU

Meat or Protein: Half of a grilled cheese sandwich (Low-fat cheese)

Carbohydrates: Two pieces of toast

Drink: Water

Fruits and Vegetables: Half a cup of strawberries

LUNCH MENU

Meat or Protein: Beef stew

Carbohydrates: Half a cup of roasted potatoes

Drink: Water and tea

Fruits and Vegetables: Black bean salad

SNACK MENU

Meat or Protein: Chicken noodle soup (low sodium type)

Carbohydrates: Cornbread

Drink: Water

Fruits and Vegetables: Green beans carrots and peas

DINNER MENU

Meat or Protein: Turkey salad with dill

Carbohydrates: Crackers

Drink: Water and white tea

Fruits and Vegetables: Three bean salad

DAY 8

EXERCISE

Daily exercise: 30 minutes on an elliptical workout machine

MORNING MENU

Meat or Protein: Half a cup of dry cereal and milk

Carbohydrates: None

Drink: Water and decaffeinated coffee

Fruits and Vegetables: One pear

SNACK MENU

Meat or Protein: Two tablespoons of cream cheese

Carbohydrates: Half a piece of toast

Drink: Water

Fruits and Vegetables: One peach

LUNCH MENU

Meat or Protein: Macaroni and cheese (One-fourth of a cup of shredded, low-fat cheese)

Carbohydrates: Half a cup of potato salad

Drink: Water and tea

Fruits and Vegetables: Salad with tomatoes, romaine lettuce, and raw yellow squash

SNACK MENU

Meat or Protein: Chicken noodle soup (Low sodium)

Carbohydrates: None

Drink: Water

Fruits and Vegetables: One apple

DINNER MENU

Meat or Protein: Grilled turkey breast

Carbohydrates: Half a cup of stuffing

Drink: Water

Fruits and Vegetables: Stewed cauliflower and low-fat cheese

DAY 9

EXERCISE

Daily exercise: Resistance step training for 30 minutes

MORNING MENU

Meat or Protein: Egg white omelet

Carbohydrates: One raspberry muffin

Drink: Decaffeinated coffee

Fruits and Vegetables: One apricot

SNACK MENU

Meat or Protein: None

Carbohydrates: Half a bagel

Drink: Water

Fruits and Vegetables: Miners lettuce, Green beans, and cantaloupe

---

LUNCH MENU

Meat or Protein: Grilled, lean pork cutlet

Carbohydrates: Half a cup of roasted potatoes

Drink: Water

Fruits and Vegetables: Green beans

SNACK MENU

Meat or Protein: None

Carbohydrates: Corn muffin

Drink: Water

Fruits and Vegetables: Two kiwis

DINNER MENU

Meat or Protein: Chickpea vegan burger

Carbohydrates: Baked zucchini

Drink: Water

Fruits and Vegetables: One cup of strawberries with plain yogurt

DAY 10

EXERCISE

Daily exercise: 30 minutes of crunches, sit-ups, push-ups and jumping jacks

MORNING MENU

Meat or Protein: Turkey bacon and egg white omelet

Carbohydrates: Blueberry pancakes

Drink: water and decaffeinated coffee

Fruits and Vegetables: Half a cup of tomato juice

Meat or Protein:

Carbohydrates: Whole grain muffin

Drink: Water

Fruits and Vegetables: Half a cup of dehydrated prunes

LUNCH MENU

Meat or Protein: Tuna salad

Carbohydrates: Half a cup of roasted potatoes

Drink: Water and tea

Fruits and Vegetables: Starfruit or an apple

SNACK MENU

Meat or Protein: Vegetable soup

Carbohydrates: Cornbread muffin

Drink: Water

Fruits and Vegetables: Blackberries

DINNER MENU

Meat or Protein: Roasted chicken thighs

Carbohydrates: Jasmine rice

Drink: Water and orange and black pekoe tea

Fruits and Vegetables: Two Oranges

DAY 11

EXERCISE

Daily exercise: Light yoga-like stretching for 20 minutes

MORNING MENU

Meat or Protein: Turkey sausage with egg white omelet

Carbohydrates: Half a cup of plain oatmeal

Drink: Water and tea

Fruits and Vegetables: One-fourth of a cup of raisins and dried cranberries

SNACK MENU

Meat or Protein: None

Carbohydrates:

Drink: Water

Fruits and Vegetables: Strawberries and peaches topped with yogurt

LUNCH MENU

Meat or Protein: Fish tacos

Carbohydrates: Tortilla

Drink: Water

Fruits and Vegetables: Two kiwis

SNACK MENU

Meat or Protein: Black beans with shredded low-fat cheddar cheese

Carbohydrates: Corn chips

Drink: Water

Fruits and Vegetables: Half a cup of blueberries and yogurt

DINNER MENU

Meat or Protein: Baked halibut

Carbohydrates: None

Drink: Water and tea

Fruits and Vegetables: Two clementine oranges

DAY 12

EXERCISE

Daily exercise: 30-minute swimming routine

MORNING MENU

Meat or Protein: Egg salad with dill

Carbohydrates: Toast

Drink: Water and tea

Fruits and Vegetables: Strawberries and blueberries with plain yogurt

---

SNACK MENU

Meat or Protein: None

Carbohydrates: Unsalted crackers

Drink: Water

Fruits and Vegetables: One pomegranate

LUNCH MENU

Meat or Protein: Baked chicken

Carbohydrates: Half a cup of roasted potatoes

Drink: Water

Fruits and Vegetables: Carrots and peas

Meat or Protein: None

Carbohydrates: One croissant

Drink: Water

Fruits and Vegetables: Two bananas

DINNER MENU

Meat or Protein: Shredded ham and low-fat cheese potatoes au gratin

Carbohydrates: Half a cup of stuffing

Drink: Water or tea

Fruits and Vegetables: Two nectarines

DAY 13

EXERCISE

Daily exercise: Brisk speed walking for half a mile

MORNING MENU

Meat or Protein: Scrambled egg whites and shredded Swiss cheese

Carbohydrates: Two slices of toast

Drink: Water and tea

Fruits and Vegetables: Strawberries and star fruit

SNACK MENU

Meat or Protein: None

Carbohydrates: Cranberry muffin

Drink: Water

Fruits and Vegetables: Fresh pineapple chunks

LUNCH MENU

Meat or Protein: Roasted pork cutlet

Carbohydrates: Half a cup of roasted potatoes

Drink: Water and green tea

Fruits and Vegetables: Two peaches

SNACK MENU

Meat or Protein: Half a cup of raw almonds

Carbohydrates: Cornbread muffin

Drink: Water

Fruits and Vegetables: Half a cup of unsalted, water-packed olives

DINNER MENU

Meat or Protein: Lamb roast

Carbohydrates: Half a cup of stuffing

Drink: Water and tea

Fruits and Vegetables: Papaya salad with papaya and tomatoes

DAY 14

EXERCISE

Daily exercise: 30 minutes of elliptical workout training on exercise bike

MORNING MENU

Meat or Protein: Scrambled egg whites and shredded low-fat cheese

Carbohydrates: One bran muffin

Drink: Decaffeinated coffee

Fruits and Vegetables One apple

SNACK MENU

Meat or Protein: None

Carbohydrates: Half of a bagel

Drink: Water

Fruits and Vegetables: Half of a cantaloupe

LUNCH MENU

Meat or Protein: Broiled veal cutlet

Carbohydrates: Half a cup of roasted potatoes

Drink: Water and tea

Fruits and Vegetables: Two kiwis

SNACK MENU

Meat or Protein: None

Carbohydrates: Cornbread

Drink: Water

Fruits and Vegetables: Two plums

DINNER MENU

Meat or Protein: Lean roasted duck breast

Carbohydrates: Half a cup of pasta

Drink: Water or tea

Fruits and Vegetables: Two tangerines

DAY 15

EXERCISE

Daily exercise: Treadmill walking for 30 minutes

MORNING MENU

Meat or Protein: Half a cup of dried cereal and milk

Carbohydrates: One bran muffin

Drink: Water and decaffeinated coffee

Fruits and Vegetables: One peach

SNACK MENU

Meat or Protein: Half a cup of pistachios

Carbohydrates: half a bagel

Drink: Water

Fruits and Vegetables: Two Oranges

LUNCH MENU

Meat or Protein: Grilled pork cutlet

Carbohydrates: Half a cup of roasted potatoes

Drink: Water and tea

Fruits and Vegetables: Half a cup of blueberries and plain yogurt

SNACK MENU

Meat or Protein: None

Carbohydrates: Raspberry muffin

Drink: Water

Fruits and Vegetables: Half a cup of dried prunes

DINNER MENU

Meat or Protein: Grilled lemon salmon

Carbohydrates: Half a cup of rice

Drink: Water or tea

Fruits and Vegetables: One apple

DAY 16

EXERCISE

Daily exercise: 30 minutes of swimming

MORNING MENU

Meat or Protein: Half a cup of plain oatmeal with blueberries

Carbohydrates: Half a bran muffin

Drinks water coffee

Fruits and Vegetables: Half a cup of strawberries and plain yogurt

SNACK MENU

Meat or Protein: Half a cup of unsalted and raw almonds

Carbohydrates ½ bagel

Drinks water

Fruits and Vegetables: Half a cantaloupe

LUNCH MENU

Meat or Protein: Turkey sandwich

Carbohydrates: Baked potato wedges

Drink: Water and orange and black pekoe tea

Fruits and Vegetables: One pomegranate

SNACK MENU

Meat or Protein: None

Carbohydrates: Dried cranberries (craisins)

Drinks water

Fruits and Vegetables: One peach

DINNER MENU

Meat or Protein: Baked beef ribs

Carbohydrates: Half a cup of pasta

Drink: Water coffee and tea

Fruits and Vegetables: Half a cup of raspberries and plain yogurt

DAY 17

EXERCISE

Daily exercise: 30 minutes of elliptical workout training on an elliptical exercise machine

MORNING MENU

Meat or Protein: Turkey sausage, eggs, and low fat shredded cheese

Carbohydrates: One English muffin

Drink: Water and decaffeinated coffee

Fruits and Vegetables: Two bananas

SNACK MENU

Meat or Protein: None

Carbohydrates: Half of a raisin bagel

Drink: Water

Fruits and Vegetables: Half a honeydew melon

LUNCH MENU

Meat or Protein: Eggplant lasagna

Carbohydrates: Half a cup of pasta

Drink: Water and tea

Fruits and Vegetables: One nectarine

SNACK MENU

Meat or Protein: None

Carbohydrates: Cornbread muffin

Drink: Water

Fruits and Vegetables: Half a cup of currants

DINNER MENU

Meat or Protein: Black bean soup with baked pork cutlet

Carbohydrates: Half a cup of soup

Drink: Water and tea

Fruits and Vegetables: Half of a honeydew melon

DAY 18

EXERCISE

Daily exercise: 30 minutes on a rowing exercise machine

MORNING MENU

Meat or Protein: Half a cup of cereal with banana slices

Carbohydrates: Two pieces of lighted butter toast

Drinks water coffee

Fruits and Vegetables: One-fourth of a cup of raisins

SNACK MENU

Meat or Protein: None

Carbohydrates: Half a bagel

Drink: Water

Fruits and Vegetables: Half a cantaloupe

LUNCH MENU

Meat or Protein: Roasted chicken breast

Carbohydrates: Half a cup of rice

Drink: Water and tea

Fruits and Vegetables: Three celery sticks with one teaspoon of salt alternative

---

SNACK MENU

Meat or Protein: None

Carbohydrates: Cornbread muffin

Drink: Water

Fruits and Vegetables: Half a cup of dried cranberries

DINNER MENU

Meat or Protein: Grilled salmon fillet

Carbohydrates: Half a cup of rice

Drink: Water and Earl Grey tea

Fruits and Vegetables: One-half cup of canned fruit cocktail (light syrup)

DAY 19

EXERCISE

Daily exercise: 30 minutes of resistance step training

MORNING MENU

Meat or Protein: Half a cup of oatmeal with sliced peaches

Carbohydrates: Two slices of lightly butter toast

Drink: Water and decaffeinated coffee

Fruits and Vegetables: One apple

SNACK MENU

Meat or Protein: One-fourth of a cup of unsalted and raw almonds

Carbohydrates: Half a bagel

Drink: Water

Fruits and Vegetables: Half a cup of strawberries and yogurt

LUNCH MENU

Meat or Protein: Chicken salad

Carbohydrates: Half a cup of roasted potatoes

Drink: Water and tea

Fruits and Vegetables: Two bananas

SNACK MENU

Meat or Protein: None

Carbohydrates: Cornbread muffin

Drink: Water

Fruits and Vegetables: Two triangle slices of watermelon

DINNER MENU

Meat or Protein: Quinoa veggie burger

Carbohydrates: Baked potato wedges

Drink: Water and tea

Fruits and Vegetables: Half a cantaloupe

DAY 20

EXERCISE

Daily exercise: Brisk walk for half a mile

MORNING MENU

Meat or Protein: Turkey bacon and egg white omelet

Carbohydrates: One English muffin

Drink: Water and coffee

Fruits and Vegetables: Half a cup of blueberries and plain yogurt

---

SNACK MENU

Meat or Protein: One-fourth of a cup of pistachios

Carbohydrates: None

Drink: Water

Fruits and Vegetables: Half a cantaloupe

LUNCH MENU

Meat or Protein: Fish tacos

Carbohydrates: Half a cup of roasted potatoes

Drink: Water and tea

Fruits and Vegetables: Two plums

SNACK MENU

Meat or Protein: None

Carbohydrates: Cornbread muffin

Drink: Water

Fruits and Vegetables: Blackberries and plain yogurt

DINNER MENU

Meat or Protein: Turkey burger

Carbohydrates: Roasted potato wedges

Drink: Water and tea

Fruits and Vegetables: Stewed broccoli

DAY 21

EXERCISE

Daily exercise: 30-minute swimming routine

MORNING MENU

Meat or Protein: Half a cup of oatmeal with blueberries

Carbohydrates: One croissant

Drink: Water and decaffeinated coffee

Fruits and Vegetables: One apricot

SNACK MENU

Meat or Protein: None

Carbohydrates: Half of a bagel

Drink: Water

Fruits and Vegetables: Half of a cantaloupe

LUNCH MENU

Meat or Protein: Tuna fish sandwich

Carbohydrates: Half a cup of pasta

Drink: Water and tea

Fruits and Vegetables: Half a cup of canned fruit cocktail

SNACK MENU

Meat or Protein: None

Carbohydrates: Blueberry bread

Drink: Water

Fruits and Vegetables: One orange

Meat or Protein: Baked halibut

Carbohydrates: Half a cup of rice

Drink: Water and tea

Fruits and Vegetables: Stewed broccoli

DAY 22

EXERCISE

Daily exercise: 30-minutes of rowing machine exercise

MORNING MENU

Meat or Protein: Turkey bacon and scrambled egg whites

Carbohydrates: One English muffin

Drink: Water and tea

Fruits and Vegetables: One-fourth of a cup of raisins

SNACK MENU

Meat or Protein: Half of a cup of unsalted and raw peanuts

Carbohydrates: One piece of toast

Drink: Water

Fruits and Vegetables: One Apple

LUNCH MENU

Meat or Protein: Fish Taco and black bean salad

Carbohydrates: Baked potato wedges

Drink: Water and tea

Fruits and Vegetables: One pear

SNACK MENU

Meat or Protein: None

Carbohydrates: Raspberry muffin

Drink: Water

Fruits and Vegetables: Half a cup of blueberries and plain yogurt

---

DINNER MENU

Meat or Protein: Grilled pork roast

Carbohydrates: Half a cup of rice

Drink: Water and tea

Fruits and Vegetables: Spinach salad

DAY 23

EXERCISE

Daily exercise: Resistance training step exercise

MORNING MENU

Meat or Protein: Half a cup of cereal with skim milk and sliced bananas

Carbohydrates: Two slices of lightly buttered toast

Drink: Water and decaffeinated coffee

Fruits and Vegetables: One apple

SNACK MENU

Meat or Protein: None

Carbohydrates: One English muffin

Drink: Water

Fruits and Vegetables: Half a honeydew melon

LUNCH MENU

Meat or Protein: Turkey sandwich

Carbohydrates: Half a cup of pasta

Drink: Water and tea

Fruits and Vegetables: One pomegranate

SNACK MENU

Meat or Protein: None

Carbohydrates: Cornbread muffin

Drink: Water

Fruits and Vegetables: Two bananas

DINNER MENU

Meat or Protein: Eggplant Lasagna

Carbohydrates: Half a cup of rice

Drink: Water and tea

Fruits and Vegetables: Cesar salad

DAY 24

EXERCISE

Daily exercise: 30-minutes of aerobic exercise

MORNING MENU

Meat or Protein: Half a cup of oatmeal with raisins

Carbohydrates: Blueberry pancakes

Drink: Water and decaffeinated coffee

Fruits and Vegetables: One apple

SNACK MENU

Meat or Protein: None

Carbohydrates One bran muffin

Drink: Water

Fruits and Vegetables: Half a cantaloupe

LUNCH MENU

Meat or Protein: Roast chicken thighs

Carbohydrates: Half a cup of roasted potatoes

Drink: Water and tea

Fruits and Vegetables: Half a cup of baby carrots

SNACK MENU

Meat or Protein: None

Carbohydrates: Cornbread muffin

Drink: Water

Fruits and Vegetables: Italian green beans

DINNER MENU

Meat or Protein: Turkey pot pie

Carbohydrates: Half a cup of pasta

Drink: Water and tea

Fruits and Vegetables: Spinach salad

DAY 25

EXERCISE

Daily exercise: Brisk power walk for half a mile

MORNING MENU

Meat or Protein: Turkey sausage and egg whites

Carbohydrates: One bran muffin

Drink: Water and coffee

Fruits and Vegetables: Half a cup of strawberries and low-fat cream

SNACK MENU

Meat or Protein: None

Carbohydrates: One croissant

Drink: Water

Fruits and Vegetables: One pear

LUNCH MENU

Meat or Protein: Tuna fish wrap

Carbohydrates: Half a cup of pasta

Drink: Water and tea

Fruits and Vegetables: One cup of grapes

SNACK MENU

Meat or Protein: None

Carbohydrates: Cornbread muffin

Drink: Water

Fruits and Vegetables: Half a cup of canned fruit cocktail

DINNER MENU

Meat or Protein: Grilled salmon fillet

Carbohydrates: Half a cup of tortellini

Drink: Water and tea

Fruits and Vegetables: Spinach salad

DAY 26

EXERCISE

Daily exercise: 30 minutes of moderate aerobic exercise

MORNING MENU

Meat or Protein: Turkey sausage and egg white omelet

Carbohydrates: One croissant

Drink: Water and decaffeinated coffee

Fruits and Vegetables: Two bananas

SNACK MENU

Meat or Protein: One-fourth of a cup of sunflower seeds

Carbohydrates: None

Drink: Water

Fruits and Vegetables: One-fourth of a cup of dried cranberries

LUNCH MENU

Meat or Protein: Roast pork

Carbohydrates: Half a cup of roasted potatoes

Drink: Water and tea

Fruits and Vegetables: Half a cup of blueberries with plain yogurt

SNACK MENU

Meat or Protein: None

Carbohydrates: Cornbread muffin

Drink: Water

Fruits and Vegetables: Pomegranate

DINNER MENU

Meat or Protein: Beef stew

Carbohydrates: Half a cup of rice

Drink: Water and tea

Fruits and Vegetables: Half a cup of canned fruit cocktail

DAY 27

EXERCISE

Daily exercise, walking, swimming, elliptical workouts some herbs that can be substituted are Hawthorne, garlic, and turmeric.

MORNING MENU

Meat or Protein: Half a cup of dry cereal and skim milk

Carbohydrates: one bran muffin

Drink: Water and coffee

Fruits and Vegetables: Two tangerines

SNACK MENU

Meat or Protein: None

Carbohydrates: One English muffin

Drink: Water

Fruits and Vegetables: One banana

LUNCH MENU

Meat or Protein: Chicken salad

Carbohydrates: Half a cup of pasta

Drink: Water and tea

Fruits and Vegetables: Spinach salad

SNACK MENU

Meat or Protein: None

Carbohydrates: One bran muffin

Drink: Water

Fruits and Vegetables: Blackberries and low-fat cream

DINNER MENU

Meat or Protein: Broiled chicken legs

Carbohydrates: Half a cup of stuffing

Drink: Water or tea

Fruits and Vegetables: Stewed broccoli

DAY 28

EXERCISE

Daily exercise: 20 minutes of swimming or 30 minutes of walking

MORNING MENU

Meat or Protein: Turkey sausage and scrambled egg whites

Carbohydrates: Two slices of lightly buttered bread

Drink: Water and decaffeinated coffee

Fruits and Vegetables: One apple

SNACK MENU

Meat or Protein: None

Carbohydrates: Half of a bagel

Drink: Water

Fruits and Vegetables: Half a honeydew melon

LUNCH MENU

Meat or Protein: Baked chicken wings

Carbohydrates: Half a cup of roasted potatoes

Drink: Water and tea

Fruits and Vegetables: Half a cup of blueberries and plain yogurt

SNACK MENU

Meat or Protein: None

Carbohydrates: Bran muffin

Drink: Water

Fruits and Vegetables: One peach

DINNER MENU

Meat or Protein: Grilled salmon fillet

Carbohydrates: Half a cup of rice

Drink: Water and tea

Fruits and Vegetables: Half a cup of canned fruit cocktail

DAY 29

EXERCISE

Daily exercise: 30-minutes of walking on a treadmill.

MORNING MENU

Meat or Protein: Low-fat cheese omelet

Carbohydrates: Raspberry muffin

Drink: Water and decaffeinated coffee

Fruits and Vegetables: One apple

SNACK MENU

Meat or Protein: One-fourth of a cup of pistachios

Carbohydrates: None

Drink: water

Fruits and Vegetables: Two watermelon triangle slices

LUNCH MENU

Meat or Protein: Crabcakes

Carbohydrates: Half a cup of pasta

Drink: Water and tea

Fruits and Vegetable: Half a cup of baby carrots

SNACK MENU

Meat or Protein: Half a cup of unsalted and raw almonds

Carbohydrates: None

Drink: Water

Fruits and Vegetables: Blackcurrants and low-fat cream

DINNER MENU

Meat or Protein: Baked halibut

Carbohydrates: Half a cup of tortellini

Drink: Water and tea

Fruits and Vegetables: Three bean salad with romaine lettuce

DAY 30

EXERCISE

Daily exercise: 30-minutes of moderate aerobic exercise

MORNING MENU

Meat or Protein: Half a cup of dry cereal with skim milk

Carbohydrates: Pancakes

Drink: Water and decaffeinated coffee

Fruits and Vegetables: One apple

SNACK MENU

Meat or Protein: None

Carbohydrates: Half a bagel

Drink: Water

Fruits and Vegetables: One banana

LUNCH MENU

Meat or Protein: Black bean soup and baked chicken strips

Carbohydrates: Half a cup of roasted potatoes

Drink: Water and tea

Fruits and Vegetable Carrots: One-half cup of canned fruit cocktail

---

SNACK MENU

Meat or Protein: None

Carbohydrates: Cornbread

Drink: Water

Fruits and Vegetables: One peach

DINNER MENU

Meat or Protein: Baked Cod

Carbohydrates: Half a cup of pasta

Drink: Water and tea

Fruits and Vegetables: Stewed carrots

DAY 31

EXERCISE

Daily exercise: 30 minutes of brisk walking for a half mile

MORNING MENU

Meat or Protein: Half a cup of oatmeal with dried cranberries

Carbohydrates: Two slices of lightly buttered toast

Drink: Water and decaffeinated coffee

Fruits and Vegetable: One apple

SNACK MENU

Meat or Protein: One-fourth of a cup of almonds

Carbohydrate: Half of a bagel

Drink: Water

Fruits and Vegetables: One apple

LUNCH MENU

Meat or Protein: Roast turkey sandwich

Carbohydrates: Baked potato wedges

Drink: Water and tea

Fruits and Vegetable: Two bananas

SNACK MENU

Meat or Protein: None

Carbohydrates: Cornbread

Drink: water

Fruits and Vegetable: Half a cup of raisin

DINNER MENU

Meat or Protein: Baked chicken

Carbohydrate: Half a cup of rice

Drink: Water and tea

Fruits and Vegetable: Green peas

Whether you have just started regularly checking your blood pressure, or have been diagnosed with high blood pressure and have had to start taking medications, there are many safe home remedies that you can try yourself. High blood pressure is a serious medical condition that should not be taken lightly.

Always get your blood pressure readings checked regularly and always follow the advice of your doctor or licensed medical professional. However, as has been mention previously in this book, it is also important to be well informed and educated high blood pressure and what you can do on your own to maintain and control. You have to educationally proactive as much as possible. This is your health, after all.

There are several natural remedies that well-researched scientific study suggests could be effective in the regular maintenance and control of high blood pressure. The use and practice of natural remedies in dealing with your high blood pressure should never take the place of advice from your doctor. It can't hurt either.

When it comes to the damage that high blood pressure can wreak on the human body, every little bit can help.

Invest in a home sphygmomanometer and get in the habit of checking your own blood pressure at home. You should trust the reading administered to you by your doctor or medical professional. However, you will have always have a rough baseline reference reading in regards to your blood pressure when you teach yourself how to check it at home.

Check out this list of scientifically recommended home remedies, ranging from teas, herbs, fruits, and spices. You should not expect to drink hibiscus tea for a week and then see your high blood pressure dramatically increase. You should use such home remedies in conjunction with adopting a healthier eating lifestyle, exercising regularly, following doctors' orders and avoiding unnecessary stress. These home remedies should not be viewed as the answer within themselves to your high blood pressure medical problems. They should be viewed as one of many tools that you can use to maintain and control your high blood pressure problems.

Here are 7 most Potent Natural Remedies to lowering your High Blood Pressure, you don't have to pick or choose between them, do them all or just a few or even just one. They are all natural foods, so they won't harm you but you may find yourself going off the medicine in just 30 days if you try them properly.

COCONUT WATER

You can get coconut water in commercial packages or in its raw form, which is best. Coconut water is the natural liquid that is found in the shell of green, unripe coconuts shells. You can buy commercially produced coconut water, but such products are usually overly processed and full of sugar. It may be best for you to buy coconut water from a trusted fruit vendor, buy unripe coconuts and extract the water yourself or buy commercially produced coconut water that is as pure as possible and minimally processed.

Natural coconut water is very rich in magnesium and potassium. Magnesium and potassium are beneficial to help regulate the function of your heart and blood vessels. It has also been suggested to help incrementally lower high blood pressure symptoms.

HIBISCUS TEA

Well researched medical studies have suggested that incorporating the use of hibiscus tea in your dietary lifestyle can help incrementally lower your high blood pressure over the long term.

Hibiscus tea acts as a natural diuretic within the human body. Of course, hibiscus tea is not as potent as the diuretic medicine that may be prescribed to you by your doctor. However, you can use hibiscus tea as a mild diuretic over the long term to help natural filter out excess sodium and fluid from your body. This will gradually and incrementally lower your blood pressure.

Some medical studies even suggest that hibiscus tea can imitate the angiotensin blocking effects of ACE inhibitor medications. ACE inhibitors are powerful high blood pressure correcting medications that are used to reverse the constricting or narrowing of arteries and blood vessels in the human body. Angiotensin is a naturally produce a bodily hormone that causes arteries, blood vessels and muscles to constrict over time. ACE inhibitors, also known as angiotensin-converting enzymes, are usually prescribed for people with severe high blood pressure problems.

Of course, hibiscus tea cannot act as a substitute for medicine prescribed by your doctor. Still, there is no harm to be done in taking long-term advantage of a low potency ACE inhibitor in the form of hibiscus tea.

GINGER-CARDAMOM TEA

Long-term scientific studies conducted by scientists in India have suggested that the regular and long-term consumption of Ginger-Cardamom tea can increase incrementally and steadily lower high blood pressure.

You will need to crush the cardamom pod seeds to release the oils within and then mix it with ginger. Put the combination on a terrycloth or sieve and then strain into a cup with hot water. Drinking Ginger-Cardamom tea for several weeks have been suggested to reduce high blood pressure, however incrementally.

FISH OIL SUPPLEMENTS

Omega-3 fatty acids, oil derived from fish, has been scientifically suggested to significantly reduce the threat of heart attacks and strokes. They have also been medically researched to show that they can incrementally reduce high blood pressure. You can find fish oil supplements over the counter at your local pharmacy. You could even talk to your doctor for recommendations.

RAW ALMONDS

Raw almonds are known for great heart health, but not many people know about their healing benefits in controlling hypertension. It is true, you should add 2-5 servings of the raw almonds to your diet every week and you will see a difference in just few weeks.

CAYENNE PEPPER

Cayenne pepper is considered to have the fastest blood pressure lowering agent in them. It is a powerful vasodilator, which means it helps expand your blood vessels which in turn helps your blood flow better and ultimately lowers your BP. But be careful consuming this hot pepper, try not to consume more than one tea spoon at a time and it is best to try it with honey or mix with other food.

RAW APPLE CIDER VINEGAR

Consumption of acetic acid (which is found in apple cider vinegar) caused a significant reduction in hypertension (high blood pressure). The research found that the acetic acid reduced blood pressure by lowering the renin activity. Renin is an enzyme which helps regulate blood pressure. I mix 1-2 table spoons in a glass of warm water in the morning.

Natural remedies do offer the benefits that you may be looking for in maintaining your high blood pressure. But any positive effects that you do experience will happen only after continued, prolonged and long-term use and not overnight. If you learn of your high blood pressure problems early enough, taking advantage of these natural remedies will be a lot more affordable than paying for potent, and in some cases very expensive, high blood pressure medications.

Additionally, if you are already taking very potent, high blood pressure medications, then using such home remedies in conjunction with your medications can't hurt either.

But remember to notify your doctor, in the event you notice seeing a lower BP rate over a longer period of time, this way your doctor can reduce or even eliminate your need for daily medicine. As a matter of fact, as I said at the beginning, that is how I got off the meds and that is how some of my family member's got off the high BP meds.

About one in three people have high blood pressure. Almost one thousand people die of high blood pressure, or complications cause by high blood pressure, every single day. Only about half of the people who have high blood pressure actually take proactive steps to maintain and reduce it. The starkest fact of all is that most people have high blood pressure and are shockingly unaware of that they have it, further endangering their lives.

High blood pressure does not reveal itself outwardly. In fact, when you realize you have high blood pressure or can recognize it manifestation within your body, that usually means that it is dangerously high and that you may be too late to reverse or reduce it by natural means or lifestyle and dietary changes.

High blood pressure is truly a silent killer. Most people do not even realize that they have it, or they realize it when it is too late.

As it has been mentioned previously in this book is the avoidable tragedy of high blood pressure. High blood pressure is avoidable. Anywhere from between sixty-seven million and seventy-five million American are living with high blood pressure, most don't even realize it, and what's worse, such a condition is avoidable.

The most important thing to remember is to be as educated and informed about your high blood pressure as possible. Get your blood pressure checked out regularly. Know your blood pressure numbers and have your doctor explain them to you. Exercise regularly. Adopt a healthier eating lifestyle. Refrain from getting stressed easily, as stress within itself can greatly increase high blood pressure over time. If you take care of your body, your body will take care of you. When you take care of your body, you are taking care of your heart. When you take care of your heart, you can maintain and normalize your blood pressure.

High blood pressure can take years or even decades before it causes enough damage to be noticeable. You have to be proactive when comes to dealing with your health, especially with your high blood pressure, and do everything that you can to maintain it and normalize it.

High blood pressure is serious but fortunately very avoidable. It is called a silent killer for a reason. However, with education and proactive steps to combat it, you can reverse or reduce your high blood pressure. You may learn about your high blood pressure early, or you may learn about it too late and need medication to maintain it.

However, it is never too late for you to do something about maintaining or reversing your high blood pressure.

Wish you a very healthy, long and happy life.

Ace Inhibitors. Medicine net. Medicinenet.com Retrieved
12/25/2017

Blood Pressure and You.
www.bloodpressureuk.org/BloodPressureandyou/Yourbody/
Enlargedheart

Blood Thinners Everyday Health. Everydayhealth.com
Retrieved 12/25/2017

Eating Well To Lower Your Blood Pressure.
http://chfs.ky.gov/NR/rdonlyres/5D24E0C9-3602-404D-
AFDC-A7195B2BDD5F/0/DASHDIET.pdf

High Blood Pressure Facts.
https://www.cdc.gov/bloodpressure/facts.htm

Know Your Risk Factors for High Blood Pressure.
www.heart.org/HEARTORG/Conditions/HighBloodPressure
/UnderstandYourRiskforHighBloodPressure/Understand-
Your-Risk-for-High-Blood-
Pressure_UCM_002052_Article.jsp#.Wljkr0xuLIU

www.ingramcontent.com/pod-product-compliance
Lightning Source LLC
Chambersburg PA
CBHW070714250726
48662CB00001B/404